Low Potassium Cookbook

50+ Smoothies, Dessert and Breakfast recipes designed for Low Potassium Diet

TABLE OF CONTENTS

BREAKFAST 7

PUMPKIN BAKED OATMEAL 7

BUCKWHEAT GRANOLA 9

FRUIT SMOOTHIE BOWL 11

BANANA PANCAKES 12

AQUAFABA GRANOLA 14

MORNING OATS 16

BANANA MUFFINS 18

CINNAMON PEANUT BUTTER 20

BANANA SPLITS 21

5 MINUTE RAW-NOLA 22

ZUCCHINI BREAD 24

PEANUT BUTTER & ACAI BOWLS 26

DARK CHOCOLATE GRANOLA 28

POTATO HASH BROWNS 30

BANANA NUT BUTTER PANCAKES 31

BREAKFAST MUFFINS 32

ZUCCHINI BANANA MUFFINS 34

GLUTEN-FREE PANCAKES 36

CINNAMON WAFFLES 37

CHEESE GRIT MUFFINS 39

CHOCHOLATE OATMEAL 41

BREAKFAST BURRITO 42

APPLE FRENCH TOAST 43

SPINACH FRITTATA 44

VEGETABLES OMELET	45
BLUEBERRY PANCAKES	47
BERRY MUFFINS	48
APPLE CRISP	50
TUNA SANDWICH	52
CHICKEN SANDWICH	53
ZUCCHINI PANCAKE	55
ZUCCHINI BREAD	57
RHUBARB CRUNCH	59
VANILLA PANCAKES	61
BREAKFAST PANCAKES	62
BUTTERMILK BISCUITS	63
APPLE CRISP	64
HAM SANDWICHES	65
CUCUMBER SANDWICHES	67
EGG TOAST	68
PEACH CRISP	69
DESSERTS	71
FRUIT BERRY SALAD	71
APPLE YOGURT PARFAIT	72
APPLE AND BLUEBERRY CRISP	73
STRAWBERRIES WITH BASIL AND BALSAMIC VINEGAR	75
LITCHI SORBET	76
BAGEL BREAD PUDDING	77
BLACK BEAN BROWNIES	78
HONEY GINGER CRACKLES	80

CRANBERRY LEMON PARFAIT 82

RICE BARS 84

SMOOTHIES 86

BANANA SMOOTHIE 86

BLUEBERRY DETOX SMOOTHIE 87

KIDNEY NOURISHING SMOOTHIE 88

CRANBERRY DETOX SMOOTHIE 89

PUMPKIN SMOOTHIE 90

CINNAMON-BLACKBERRY SMOOTHIE 91

KALE LIVER DETOX SMOOTHIE 92

GREEN DETOX SMOOTHIE 93

CLEANSE JUICE 94

CARROT AND APPLE MORNING SMOOTHIE 95

ENERGY BOOSTING SMOOTHIE 96

PAPAYA SMOOTHIE 97

NO MILK SHAKE 98

TURMERIC SMOOTHIE 99

BEETROOT DETOX SMOOTHIE 100

CARROT & BEETROOT SMOOTHIE 101

SPINACH SMOOTHIE 102

PEACH SMOOTHIE 103

GRAPEFRUIT SMOOTHIE 104

KIWI SMOOTHIE 105

☞Copyright 2018 by Noah Jerris - All rights reserved.

This document is geared towards providing exact and reliable information in regards to the topic and issue covered. The publication is sold with the idea that the publisher is not required to render accounting, officially permitted, or otherwise, qualified services. If advice is necessary, legal or professional, a practiced individual in the profession should be ordered.

- From a Declaration of Principles which was accepted and approved equally by a Committee of the American Bar Association and a Committee of Publishers and Associations.

In no way is it legal to reproduce, duplicate, or transmit any part of this document in either electronic means or in printed format. Recording of this publication is strictly prohibited and any storage of this document is not allowed unless with written permission from the publisher. All rights reserved.

The information provided herein is stated to be truthful and consistent, in that any liability, in terms of inattention or otherwise, by any usage or abuse of any policies, processes, or directions contained within is the solitary and utter responsibility of the recipient reader. Under no circumstances will any legal responsibility or blame be held against the publisher for any reparation, damages, or monetary loss due to the information herein, either directly or indirectly.

Respective authors own all copyrights not held by the publisher.

The information herein is offered for informational purposes solely, and is universal as so. The presentation of the information is without contract or any type of guarantee assurance.

The trademarks that are used are without any consent, and the publication of the trademark is without permission or backing by the trademark owner. All trademarks and brands within this book are for clarifying purposes only and are the owned by the owners themselves, not affiliated with this document.

Introduction

Low potassium recipes for personal enjoyment but also for family enjoyment. You will love them for sure for how easy it is to prepare them.

BREAKFAST

PUMPKIN BAKED OATMEAL

Serves: **6**

Prep Time: **10** Minutes

Cook Time: **30** Minutes

Total Time: **40** Minutes

INGREDIENTS

- ½ cup pumpkin puree
- 2 batches flax eggs
- 1/3 cup maple syrup
- 2 tablespoons coconut oil
- ½ tsp salt
- 1 tsp pumpkin pie spice
- ¼ tsp cinnamon
- 2 cups dairy-free milk
- 2 cups gluten-free rolled oats
- 1/3 cup pecans
- 1/3 cup frozen cranberries
- 2 tablespoons coconut sugar

DIRECTIONS

1. Preheat the oven to 325 F
2. In a bowl prepare flax eggs, add pumpkin puree, salt, maple syrup, oil, pumpkin pie spice, cinnamon and whisk to combine
3. Add milk, pecans, oats and stir to combine
4. Transfer to a baking dish and top with pecans
5. Sprinkle with coconut sugar and cranberries
6. Bake for 30-35 minutes or until golden brown
7. When ready remove and serve

BUCKWHEAT GRANOLA

Serves: **18**

Prep Time: **10** Minutes

Cook Time: **30** Minutes

Total Time: **40** Minutes

INGREDIENTS

- **1 cup buckwheat groats**
- **1 cup gluten-free oats**
- **1/3 cup raw nuts**
- **¼ cup unsweetened coconut flakes**
- **2 tablespoons chia seeds**
- **2 tablespoons coconut sugar**
- **¼ tsp salt**
- **1/3 ground cinnamon**
- **¼ cup olive oil**
- **¼ cup maple syrup**
- **2 tablespoons seed butter**
- **½ cup dried fruit**

DIRECTIONS

1. Preheat the oven to 325 F
2. In a bowl add oats, nuts, buckwheat groats, coconut, coconut sugar, chia seeds, cinnamon and salt
3. In a saucepan add olive oil, maple syrup, nut butter and pour over the dry ingredients and mix well
4. Spread the mixture evenly onto a baking sheet and bake for 25-28 minutes
5. Add dried fruits and store in the refrigerator

FRUIT SMOOTHIE BOWL

Serves: **3**

Prep Time: **5** Minutes

Cook Time: **5** Minutes

Total Time: **10** Minutes

INGREDIENTS

- 2 packets frozen dragon fruit
- ¼ cup frozen raspberries
- 2 bananas
- 2 tablespoons protein powder
- ½ cup dairy-free milk

DIRECTIONS

1. **In a blender add all ingredients and blend until smooth**
2. **Adjust flavor by adding more banana or dairy-free milk**
3. **Divide between serving bowl and top with granola and serve**

BANANA PANCAKES

Serves: **4**

Prep Time: **10** Minutes

Cook Time: **15** Minutes

Total Time: **25** Minutes

INGREDIENTS

- ¼ cup coconut flour
- 1 banana
- ¼ cup water
- 1 egg
- 1 tablespoon honey
- 1 tsp cinnamon
- ¼ tsp baking soda
- ½ tsp salt
- ¼ tablespoon vanilla extract
- 1 tablespoon coconut oil

DIRECTIONS

1. Place all ingredients in a bowl and mix using a hand mixer
2. In a skillet add coconut oil and pour ¼ cup batter

3. Cook for 1-2 minutes per side
4. When ready remove and serve with syrup

AQUAFABA GRANOLA

Serves: **12**

Prep Time: **10** Minutes

Cook Time: **25** Minutes

Total Time: **35** Minutes

INGREDIENTS

- 2 cups gluten-free rolled oats
- 1 cup chopped raw nuts
- ¼ cup shredded coconut
- 1 tablespoon chia seeds
- ½ cup coconut sugar
- ¼ tsp salt
- ¼ tsp cinnamon
- ½ cup aquafaba
- ½ cup maple syrup
- 1 tsp vanilla extract
- ½ cup blueberries

DIRECTIONS

1. **Preheat oven to 325 F**

2. In a bowl add oats, nuts, chia seeds, coconut, coconut sugar, cinnamon, salt and stir to combine
3. Add aquafaba to a mixing bowl and use a hand mixer
4. Add maple syrup and vanilla and pour aquafaba mixture over the dry ingredients
5. Spread the mixture onto a parchment paper and bake for 30-35 minutes
6. Add dried fruits and serve when ready

MORNING OATS

Serves: **2**

Prep Time: **10** Minutes

Cook Time: **15** Minutes

Total Time: **25** Minutes

INGREDIENTS

- 1 cup oats
- 2 cup water
- 1 pinch salt
- 1 tablespoon flaxseed meal
- 1 tablespoon maple syrup
- ½ tsp ground cinnamon
- fruit compote

DIRECTIONS

1. In a saucepan add water, oats, cover and soak for 4-5 hours or overnight
2. Add a pinch of salt and bring to a boil
3. Reduce heat and cook for 10-12 minutes or until the water is almost absorbed
4. When they are ready remove from heat

5. Divide between serving bowl, top with chia seeds, banana, almond milk and serve

BANANA MUFFINS

Serves: **12**

Prep Time: **10** Minutes

Cook Time: **30** Minutes

Total Time: **40** Minutes

INGREDIENTS

- 1 cup almond flour
- 1 cup pecan pieces
- 1 tsp cinnamon
- ¼ tsp nutmeg
- ¼ tsp baking powder
- ½ tsp salt
- 2 bananas
- 1 tablespoon honey
- 2 eggs

DIRECTIONS

1. **Preheat the oven to 400 F**
2. **In a food processor add pecan pieces, cinnamon, almond flour, nutmeg, baking powder, salt and process for 45-60 seconds**

3. Mush bananas, add honey, eggs and mix well
4. Add the flour mixture to the egg mixture and mix well
5. Scoop the butter into 12 muffin cups
6. Bake for 22-25 minutes or until ready

CINNAMON PEANUT BUTTER

Serves: **12**

Prep Time: **10** Minutes

Cook Time: **10** Minutes

Total Time: **20** Minutes

INGREDIENTS

- 2 cups unsalted peanuts
- ½ tsp salt
- 2 tablespoons cinnamon
- ½ tsp powdered stevia
- 1 tablespoon avocado oil
- ½ cup raisins

DIRECTIONS

1. **In a blender add peanuts and blend for 4-5 minutes**
2. **Add cinnamon, salt, sweetener and blend for another 30-60 seconds**
3. **Add raisins and blend for another 30 seconds**
4. **Add more cinnamon if necessary and serve**

BANANA SPLITS

Serves: **4**

Prep Time: **5** Minutes

Cook Time: **5** Minutes

Total Time: **10** Minutes

INGREDIENTS

- 4 bananas
- ¼ cup nut butter
- ½ cup coconut yogurt
- ½ cup Rawnola
- ¼ cup berries
- 3 tsp hemp seeds
- ½ cup unsweetened coconut flakes

DIRECTIONS

1. Cut a slit down the center of each banana
2. Top with nut butter, rawnola, berries, coconut yogurt, hemp seeds and coconut flakes
3. When ready, serve fresh

5 MINUTE RAW-NOLA

Serves: **4**

Prep Time: **10** Minutes

Cook Time: **45** Minutes

Total Time: **55** Minutes

INGREDIENTS

- 1 cup raw walnuts
- 14-16 pitted dates
- 1 heaping tablespoon hemp seeds
- 1 heaping tablespoon flaxseed meal
- 1 tsp chia seeds
- ¼ cup unsweetened coconut
- ¼ cup gluten-free oats
- ¼ tsp cinnamon
- ¼ tsp maca powder
- 1 pinch salt
- 2 tablespoons cacao ribs
- ½ cup cacao powder
- 1 tsp vanilla extract

DIRECTIONS

1. In a blender add nuts, dates and blend for 5-6 minutes
2. Add remaining ingredients and mix well
3. Add cacao ribs, dried fruits, vanilla extract and cacao powder
4. Blend again, top with coconut yogurt and enjoy

ZUCCHINI BREAD

Serves: **12**

Prep Time: **10** Minutes

Cook Time: **60** Minutes

Total Time: **70** Minutes

INGREDIENTS

- 2 batches flax egg
- ½ cup applesauce
- ½ cup maple syrup
- ½ cup coconut sugar
- 1 tsp baking soda
- 1 tsp baking powder
- ½ tsp salt
- ¼ cup unsweetened cocoa powder
- ½ cup melted coconut oil
- ½ cup unsweetened almond milk
- 1 cup zucchini
- 1/3 cup gluten-free flour blend
- ½ cup almond flour
- ½ cup chocolate chips

DIRECTIONS

1. Preheat the oven to 350 F
2. In a bowl mix flax eggs add maple syrup, coconut sugar, applesauce, baking soda, baking powder, cocoa powder, salt and whisk well
3. Add coconut oil, almond milk, grated zucchini and stir to combine
4. Add out flour, almond flour, and stir in chocolate chips
5. Transfer batter to the loaf pan and top with a couple of chocolate chips
6. Bake for 45-55 minutes or until done
7. When ready remove and serve

PEANUT BUTTER & ACAI BOWLS

Serves: **4**

Prep Time: **10** Minutes

Cook Time: **15** Minutes

Total Time: **25** Minutes

INGREDIENTS

- 2 packets unsweetened acai
- 1 banana
- 2 tablespoons peanut butter powder
- ½ cup unsweetened coconut
- 1 cup spinach
- ½ cup mixed berries

TOPPINGS

- ½ banana
- 1 tablespoon unsweetened coconut
- 2 tablespoons sunflower seeds

DIRECTIONS

1. In a blender add acai, dairy-free milk, peanut butter powder, spinach and blend until smooth

2. Blend until the mixture is thick
3. Adjust flavor by adding peanut butter powder
4. Divide between 2 serving bowls garnish with toppings and serve

DARK CHOCOLATE GRANOLA

Serves: 8
Prep Time: 10   Minutes
Cook Time: 25   Minutes
Total Time: 35   Minutes

INGREDIENTS

- 2 cups gluten free rolled oats
- 1 cup chopped raw nuts
- ½ cup shredded coconut
- 2 tablespoons chia seeds
- 2 tablespoons coconut sugar
- 1 tsp salt
- ½ cup cocoa powder
- ½ cup coconut oil
- ¼ cup maple syrup
- ¼ cup dark chocolate chips

DIRECTIONS

1. Preheat the oven to 350 F

2. In a blender add coconut, chia seeds, nuts, oats, salt, coconut sugar and cocoa powder and blend until smooth
3. In a saucepan add coconut oil, maple syrup and pour melted mixture over the dry ingredients and mix well
4. Spread the mixture onto a baking sheet and bake for 20-25 minutes or until golden brown
5. When ready remove from the oven and serve

POTATO HASH BROWNS

Serves: **4**

Prep Time: **10** Minutes

Cook Time: **20** Minutes

Total Time: **30** Minutes

INGREDIENTS

- 2 sweet potatoes
- 1 tablespoon avocado oil
- 1 pinch of salt
- 1 pinch of pepper

DIRECTIONS

1. **Spiralize your potatoes into thin noodles**
2. **In a skillet add olive oil, sweet potatoes and season with salt and pepper**
3. **Cook for 8-10 minutes or until crispy**
4. **When ready, serve with herbs or hot sauce**

BANANA NUT BUTTER PANCAKES

Serves: **4**

Prep Time: **10** Minutes

Cook Time: **20** Minutes

Total Time: **30** Minutes

INGREDIENTS

- 2 bananas
- ¼ cup pecan butter
- 3 eggs
- 1 tsp baking soda

DIRECTIONS

1. In a bowl mix all pancake ingredients
2. Pour batter in a greased skillet
3. Cook for 1-2 minutes per side and serve with strawberry syrup

BREAKFAST MUFFINS

Serves: **2**

Prep Time: **10** Minutes

Cook Time: **30** Minutes

Total Time: **40** Minutes

INGREDIENTS

- 2 eggs
- ½ cup yogurt
- 2 tablespoons olive oil
- ¼ lb. apple sauce
- 1 banana
- 3 tablespoons honey
- 1 tsp vanilla extract
- ½ lb. whole meal flour
- 2 oz. oats
- 1 tsp baking powder
- 1 tsp cinnamon
- ¼ lb. blueberry

DIRECTIONS

1. **Preheat oven to 300 F**

2. In a bowl mix all ingredients
3. Pour batter into 12 large muffin cases
4. Sprinkle with extra oats and seeds
5. Bake for 22-25 minutes or until golden brown
6. When ready remove and serve

ZUCCHINI BANANA MUFFINS

Serves: **4**

Prep Time: **10** Minutes

Cook Time: **15** Minutes

Total Time: **25** Minutes

INGREDIENTS

- 2 bananas
- 1 zucchini
- 1 egg
- ½ cup nut butter
- 1 tsp cinnamon
- ¾ shredded unsweetened coconut
- ¼ cup almond flour
- ¼ tsp salt

DIRECTIONS

1. Preheat the oven to 350 F
2. In a bowl mash the bananas
3. Add grated zucchini, egg, nut butter and mix well
4. Stir in coconut, almond flour, salt, cinnamon, and mix well

5. Fill each muffin tin with a ¼ cup of the mixture
6. Bake for 12-15 minutes
7. When ready, remove and serve

GLUTEN-FREE PANCAKES

Serves: **6**

Prep Time: **10** Minutes

Cook Time: **10** Minutes

Total Time: **20** Minutes

INGREDIENTS

- 1 cup gluten-free flour blend
- 1 cup buttermilk
- 1 egg
- 1 tablespoon sugar
- 2 tablespoons unsalted butter
- 2 tsp gluten-free baking powder
- ½ tsp salt
- maple syrup

DIRECTIONS

1. In a bowl mix all ingredients until smooth
2. Heat a griddle to 325 F
3. Spoon ¼ cup batter onto griddle and cook for 1-2 minutes per side
4. When ready remove and serve with syrup

CINNAMON WAFFLES

Serves: 5
Prep Time: 10 Minutes
Cook Time: 20 Minutes
Total Time: 30 Minutes

INGREDIENTS

- 1 cup low-fat yogurt
- ½ cup nonfat milk
- 1 egg
- 1 tablespoon honey
- 1 tablespoon butter
- 1 cup whole wheat flour
- 2 tsp baking powder
- 1 tsp cinnamon

DIRECTIONS

1. Preheat waffle iron
2. In a bowl mix all ingredients for the waffles
3. Pour ¼ cup batter into waffle iron and cook according to the instructions

4. When ready remove and serve with maple syrup or honey

CHEESE GRIT MUFFINS

Serves: **12**

Prep Time: **15** Minutes

Cook Time: **45** Minutes

Total Time: **60** Minutes

INGREDIENTS

- 1 cup all-purpose flour
- 1 tsp baking powder
- ¼ tsp baking soda
- ¼ tsp salt
- 1 egg
- 1/3 cup buttermilk
- ½ cup butter
- 1 cup grits
- 1 cup grated cheddar cheese
- 1 tablespoon fresh chives

DIRECTIONS

1. Preheat oven to 325 F and grease a 12 cups of muffin pan with butter
2. In a bowl mix all ingredients for muffins

3. Stir in cheese, chives and spoon batter into muffin cups
4. Bake for 30 minutes or until muffins are golden brown
5. When ready, remove and serve

CHOCHOLATE OATMEAL

Serves: **3**

Prep Time: **10** Minutes

Cook Time: **25** Minutes

Total Time: **35** Minutes

INGREDIENTS

- 1 cup low-fat yogurt
- ½ cup low-fat chocolate milk
- 1 tablespoon creamy peanut butter
- 1 cup oat-fashioned oats
- ¼ cup strawberries

DIRECTIONS

1. In a bowl combine chocolate milk, peanut butter, oats, yogurt and stir well
2. Divide mixture among 4 serving size containers
3. Top with strawberries and serve

BREAKFAST BURRITO

Serves: **1**

Prep Time: **5** Minutes

Cook Time: **10** Minutes

Total Time: **15** Minutes

INGREDIENTS

- 2 tbs salsa
- 4 eggs
- 4 tbs green chilies
- ½ tsp cumin
- 1 tsp hot pepper sauce
- 2 tortillas

DIRECTIONS

1. Grease a skillet with butter
2. Whisk the eggs in a bowl with the green chilies, hot sauce and cumin
3. Cook in the skillet until done
4. Heat the tortillas for 15 seconds
5. Spread the eggs onto the tortillas and roll up
6. Serve with salsa

APPLE FRENCH TOAST

Serves: 2
Prep Time: 5 Minutes
Cook Time: 10 Minutes
Total Time: 15 Minutes

INGREDIENTS

- 4 slices bread
- 2 eggs
- ¼ tsp mint
- ½ cup milk
- 1 cup apple sauce

DIRECTIONS

1. Mix well the ingredients in a bowl
2. Dip the bread slices in the mixture
3. Fry until gold on both sides

SPINACH FRITTATA

Serves: **6**

Prep Time: **10** Minutes

Cook Time: **10** Minutes

Total Time: **20** Minutes

INGREDIENTS

- 1 cup cheese
- 1 clove garlic
- 2 cups spinach
- 2 eggs
- 1 tbs herbs
- 2 tbs olive oil
- 1 onion

DIRECTIONS

1. **Preheat the oven to 350F**
2. **Sauté the onion and garlic in the olive oil**
3. **Add the spinach and sauté until it wilts**
4. **Mix the cheese, eggs and herbs in a bowl**
5. **Add the egg mixture in the pan**
6. **Cook in the oven for 10 minutes**

VEGETABLES OMELET

Serves: *1*

Prep Time: *5* Minutes

Cook Time: *10* Minutes

Total Time: *15* Minutes

INGREDIENTS

- 1 egg
- 1 ½ oz cheese
- 1/3 cup corn
- 1/3 tsp black pepper
- 1/3 cup zucchini
- 4 tbs green onion
- 2 tbs water
- 2 egg whites

DIRECTIONS

1. Sauté the onions, zucchini, and corn in a coated pan until tender
2. Mix the egg, egg whites, pepper and water in a bowl
3. Pour in a pan and cook for 3 minutes
4. Spread the vegetables and cheese over

5. Fold in half and cook until done
6. Serve immediately

BLUEBERRY PANCAKES

Serves: **12**
Prep Time: **10** Minutes
Cook Time: **10** Minutes
Total Time: **20** Minutes

INGREDIENTS

- 2 eggs
- 1 ½ tbs baking powder
- 3 tbs sugar
- 1 cup buttermilk
- 1 cup blueberries
- 1 ½ cups flour
- 2 ½ tbs margarine

DIRECTIONS

1. Combine the flour, sugar and baking powder in a bowl
2. Add the remaining ingredients in a well in the center
3. Stir gradually to form a smooth batter
4. Spoon out pancakes, cook until done

BERRY MUFFINS

Serves: **12**

Prep Time: **10** Minutes

Cook Time: **20** Minutes

Total Time: **30** Minutes

INGREDIENTS

- 1 cup flour
- ¾ cup blueberries
- 2/3 cup brown sugar
- 1 lemon
- 1 ½ tbs lemon juice
- ¾ cup raspberries
- ½ tsp baking soda
- 2 eggs
- ½ cup applesauce
- ¼ cup canola oil
- 1 orange
- ½ cup oatmeal

DIRECTIONS

1. Preheat the oven to 350F
2. Line 12 muffin cups with paper
3. Mix the oatmeal, flour, brown sugar, and baking soda
4. Mix together the wet ingredients
5. Stir in the dry ingredients, then add the berries
6. Scoop into the muffin cups
7. Bake for 20 minutes
8. Allow to cool, then serve

APPLE CRISP

Serves: *8*

Prep Time: *10* Minutes

Cook Time: *50* Minutes

Total Time: *60* Minutes

INGREDIENTS
Crisp
- ¼ cup flour
- 6 tbs margarine
- 1 ¼ cups oats
- ¼ cup brown sugar

Filling
- 2 cups apples
- ½ cup brown sugar
- 4 tsp cornstarch
- 4 cups blueberries
- 1 tbs margarine
- ½ tbs lemon juice

DIRECTIONS

1. **Preheat the oven to 350F**

2. Mix the dry ingredients, stir in the butter, then set aside
3. Mix the brown sugar and cornstarch
4. Add the fruits and lemon juice
5. Top with the crisp mixture and bake for 50 minutes
6. Serve warm

TUNA SANDWICH

Serves: *1*

Prep Time: *5* Minutes

Cook Time: *5* Minutes

Total Time: *10* Minutes

INGREDIENTS

- 1 leaf lettuce
- 2 slices bread
- ¼ can tuna
- 1 tbs mayonnaise

DIRECTIONS

1. Strain and rinse the tuna
2. Mix the tuna with the mayonnaise
3. Spread over the bread
4. Top with lettuce and serve

CHICKEN SANDWICH

Serves: 2
Prep Time: 5 Minutes
Cook Time: 5 Minutes
Total Time: 10 Minutes

INGREDIENTS

- 2 slices bread
- 1 grilled chicken breast
- Basil leaves
- ½ cup grapes
- 1 green onion
- ½ cup celery
- 1 tbs mayonnaise
- 2-pieces leaf lettuce
- 1 tbs lemon juice
- ¼ tsp cinnamon

DIRECTIONS

1. Mix the chicken, grapes and celery in a bowl
2. Combine the mayonnaise, cinnamon and lemon juice
3. Stir and spread over toast

4. Top with lettuce leaf
5. Add the remaining dressing to the chicken
6. Spoon the mixture over the lettuce
7. Serve garnished with basil leaves

ZUCCHINI PANCAKE

Serves: **12**

Prep Time: **5** Minutes

Cook Time: **10** Minutes

Total Time: **15** Minutes

INGREDIENTS

- 2 tbs cilantro
- ½ tsp black pepper
- 1 cup flour
- 1 cup corn
- 1 tsp baking soda
- ½ tsp cumin
- 3 eggs
- 1 tbs white sugar
- 2 zucchini
- 2 tbs oil
- ½ cup milk

DIRECTIONS

1. Mix the eggs, milk, oil, flour, baking soda, and sugar
2. Fold in corn, zucchini and spices

3. Coat a skillet
4. Cook the batter until golden
5. Serve warm

ZUCCHINI BREAD

Serves: **24**

Prep Time: **10** Minutes

Cook Time: **50** Minutes

Total Time: **60** Minutes

INGREDIENTS

- 1 cup oil
- 1 tsp salt
- 1 tsp baking powder
- 1 tbs cinnamon
- 3 eggs
- 1 tsp baking soda
- 2 ¼ cups white sugar
- 3 tsp vanilla
- 2 cups zucchini
- 1 cup walnuts
- 3 cups flour

DIRECTIONS

1. Preheat the oven to 325F
2. Sift flour, cinnamon, baking powder, and soda in a bowl
3. Whisk the oil, eggs, sugar and vanilla in a bowl
4. Stir in the flour mixture
5. Add the zucchini and nuts
6. Pour the batter into a greased pan
7. Bake for 50 minutes
8. Allow to cool, then serve

RHUBARB CRUNCH

Serves: **18**
Prep Time: **10**   Minutes
Cook Time: **50**   Minutes
Total Time: **60**   Minutes

INGREDIENTS

- 1 cup sugar
- 3 tbs flour
- 1 cup brown sugar
- 1 cup butter
- 1 cup oats
- 4 cups strawberries
- 3 cups rhubarb
- 2 cups flour

DIRECTIONS

1. **Preheat the oven to 375F**
2. **Mix the strawberries, sugar, rhubarb, and 3 tbs flour in a bowl**
3. **Mix 1 ½ cups flour, butter, oats, and brown sugar until crumbly**

4. Place on top of the fruit mixture
5. Bake for 50 minutes
6. Serve immediately

VANILLA PANCAKES

Serves: **2**

Prep Time: **5** Minutes

Cook Time: **10** Minutes

Total Time: **15** Minutes

INGREDIENTS

- 2 tbs cinnamon
- ¼ cup flour
- 3 eggs
- 2 tbs vanilla
- 2 tbs butter
- ½ cup water
- 3 tsp Splenda

DIRECTIONS

1. Mix all of the ingredients in a bowl, except for the butter, and adding the flour last
2. Pour the batter in the butter greased pan
3. Cook until golden
4. Serve immediately

BREAKFAST PANCAKES

Serves: **2**

Prep Time: **10** Minutes

Cook Time: **10** Minutes

Total Time: **20** Minutes

INGREDIENTS

- 1 egg
- 1 cup milk
- 1/8 tsp baking soda
- 2 tbs sugar
- 1 cup flour

DIRECTIONS

1. Mix the ingredients well to form a batter
2. Cook the batter in a skillet until golden on both sides
3. Serve immediately

BUTTERMILK BISCUITS

Serves: *8*

Prep Time: *5* Minutes

Cook Time: *10* Minutes

Total Time: *15* Minutes

INGREDIENTS

- 2 tsp sugar
- 1 tsp baking powder
- 4 tbs butter
- ½ cup buttermilk
- 1 ½ cups flour

DIRECTIONS

1. **Mix the dry ingredients together**
2. **Cut the butter**
3. **Add the buttermilk to form a dough**
4. **Cut the dough into biscuits**
5. **Bake at 350F for 10 minutes**

APPLE CRISP

Serves: **8**

Prep Time: **15** Minutes

Cook Time: **45** Minutes

Total Time: **60** Minutes

INGREDIENTS

- ½ cup butter
- 1 cup brown sugar
- 3 cups apples
- ½ cup sugar
- 2 tsp cinnamon
- 1 cup oats
- 1 cup flour

DIRECTIONS

1. **Preheat the oven to 350F**
2. **Mix all of the ingredients, except for the apples, in a bowl**
3. **Spread the apples over the crumb mixture and top with sugar, cinnamon and crumb mixture**
4. **Bake for 45 minutes**

HAM SANDWICHES

Serves: **24**

Prep Time: **10** Minutes

Cook Time: **20** Minutes

Total Time: **30** Minutes

INGREDIENTS

- 1 tbs poppy seeds
- ¾ cup butter
- 1 ½ tbs onion
- 24 sandwich rolls
- 1 lb cooked ham
- 1 lb cheese
- 2 tbs Dijon mustard
- 2 tsp Worcestershire sauce

DIRECTIONS

1. Preheat the oven to 350F
2. Mix the mustard, sauce, butter, onion and poppy seeds in a bowl
3. Layer half of the ham on the bottom side of the rolls in baking dish

4. Place cheese on top, then add the remaining ham
5. Place the top of the rolls on top
6. Pour the mustard mixture over
7. Bake for 20 minutes
8. Serve hot

CUCUMBER SANDWICHES

Serves: **30**

Prep Time: **10** Minutes

Cook Time: **30** Minutes

Total Time: **40** Minutes

INGREDIENTS

- 1 pinch dill weed
- 8 oz cream cheese
- ½ cup mayonnaise
- 7 oz salad dressing mix
- 2 loaves French bread
- 2 cucumbers

DIRECTIONS

1. Mix the cream cheese, dressing mix and mayonnaise in a bowl
2. Refrigerate overnight
3. Spread over the bread slices
4. Top with cucumber slices
5. Sprinkle with dill
6. Serve immediately

EGG TOAST

Serves: **1**

Prep Time: **1** Minutes

Cook Time: **4** Minutes

Total Time: **5** Minutes

INGREDIENTS

- 1 egg
- Salt
- Pepper
- 1 slice bread
- 1 tsp bacon grease

DIRECTIONS

1. Melt the bacon grease in a pan
2. Cut a circle in the middle of the bread slice
3. Lay in the pan and cook for 2 minutes
4. Flip and crack the egg in the hole
5. Season and cook until done
6. Serve hot

PEACH CRISP

Serves: **8**

Prep Time: **10** Minutes

Cook Time: **30** Minutes

Total Time: **40** Minutes

INGREDIENTS

- ½ cup brown sugar
- ½ cup butter
- 2 tsp cinnamon
- ½ tsp salt
- 1 cup oats
- 4 cups peaches
- ½ cup flour

DIRECTIONS

1. Preheat the oven to 350F
2. Arrange the peaches in a baking dish
3. Mix the ingredients together and sprinkle over the peaches
4. Press down a little and bake until golden
5. Serve immediately

DESSERTS

FRUIT BERRY SALAD

Serves: **2**

Prep Time: **5** Minutes

Cook Time: **5** Minutes

Total Time: **10** Minutes

INGREDIENTS

- 1 cup cherries
- 1 cup blackberries
- 1 cup raspberries
- 1 cup blueberries
- 1 tablespoon honey
- 1 serving yogurt cream

DIRECTIONS

1. In a bowl combine honey and berries
2. In another bowl pour yogurt cream
3. Spread yogurt cream on each plate and garnish with berry fruit salad

APPLE YOGURT PARFAIT

Serves: **4**

Prep Time: **10** Minutes

Cook Time: **10** Minutes

Total Time: **20** Minutes

INGREDIENTS

- 1 apple
- 1 cup bran flakes
- 1 cup low-fat yogurt

DIRECTIONS

1. In a glass add yogurt, cup brand flakes and apples
2. Top with yogurt and sprinkle with cinnamon
3. Serve when ready

APPLE AND BLUEBERRY CRISP

Serves: **6**

Prep Time: **10** Minutes

Cook Time: **60** Minutes

Total Time: **70** Minutes

INGREDIENTS

- 1 cup quick-cooking oats
- ½ cup brown sugar
- ½ cup all-purpose flour
- 5 tablespoons margarine

FILLING

- ¼ cup brown sugar
- 3 tsp cornstarch
- 3 cups blueberries
- 2 cups chopped apples
- 1 tablespoon margarine
- 1 tablespoon lemon juice

DIRECTIONS

1. **Preheat the oven to 325 F**

2. In a bowl mix all ingredients and mix well
3. In a baking dish mix cornstarch and brown sugar
4. Add fruits, lemon juice and toss well
5. Top with crisp mixture
6. Bake for 50-60 minutes or until golden brown
7. When ready remove and serve

STRAWBERRIES WITH BASIL AND BALSAMIC VINEGAR

Serves: **6**

Prep Time: **10** Minutes

Cook Time: **30** Minutes

Total Time: **40** Minutes

INGREDIENTS

- ½ cup sugar
- ½ cup balsamic vinegar
- 1 tablespoon honey
- ¼ tsp black pepper
- 1 tablespoon basil leaves
- 2 cups strawberries

DIRECTIONS

1. In a bowl stir together honey, pepper, vinegar and sugar
2. Add strawberries, basil and toss to coat
3. Let it chill for 30-60 minutes
4. Cut into 6-8 portions and serve with strawberries

LITCHI SORBET

Serves: **4**

Prep Time: **10** Minutes

Cook Time: **180** Minutes

Total Time: **190** Minutes

INGREDIENTS

- 1 can litchis
- 1 tablespoon powdered sugar
- 1 pasteurized egg white
- sliced lemon wedge

DIRECTIONS

1. In a blender add litchi, sugar and blend until smooth
2. Press the puree through a strainer
3. Freeze for 2-3 hours
4. Place the mixture black in the blender add the egg white and blend again
5. Return mixture to a container and freeze overnight

BAGEL BREAD PUDDING

Serves: **8**

Prep Time: **10** Minutes

Cook Time: **30** Minutes

Total Time: **40** Minutes

INGREDIENTS

- 1 bagel
- 1 cup milk
- ¼ cup egg product
- ¼ cup sugar
- 1 tsp cinnamon

DIRECTIONS

1. Break bagel into small pieces and place in a baking dish
2. In a bowl mix together egg product, sugar, cinnamon, milk and pour over bagel pieces and set aside
3. Place in the oven and bake for 25-30 minutes or until brown
4. When ready remove and serve

BLACK BEAN BROWNIES

Serves: **12**

Prep Time: **5** Minutes

Cook Time: **15** Minutes

Total Time: **20** Minutes

INGREDIENTS

- 1 can black beans
- 1 tablespoon cocoa powder
- ¼ cup oats
- ½ tsp salt
- ¼ cup maple syrup
- ½ cup coconut oil
- 1 tsp vanilla extract
- ¼ tsp baking powder
- ¼ cup chocolate chips

DIRECTIONS

1. **Preheat oven to 325 F**
2. **In a blender add all ingredients and blend until smooth**
3. **Stir in chocolate chips and pour mixture into a pan**

4. Bake for 20-25 minutes or until olden brown
5. When ready remove from the oven and serve

HONEY GINGER CRACKLES

Serves: **24**

Prep Time: **10** Minutes

Cook Time: **10** Minutes

Total Time: **20** Minutes

INGREDIENTS

- ¾ cup shortening
- 1 cup sugar
- 1 egg
- ½ cup honey
- 2 cups all-purpose flour
- 1 tsp baking soda
- 2 tsp ginger
- 1 tsp cinnamon
- 1 tsp ground cloves

DIRECTIONS

1. Preheat oven to 350 F
2. In a bowl cream together wet ingredients with dry ingredients, mix well
3. Drop in heaping tablespoons into granulated sugar

4. Roll small balls and place on a cookie sheet
5. Bake for 10-12 minutes
6. When ready remove and serve

CRANBERRY LEMON PARFAIT

Serves: **12**

Prep Time: **10** Minutes

Cook Time: **50** Minutes

Total Time: **60** Minutes

INGREDIENTS

CRANBERRY COMPOTE
- ½ lb. cranberries
- 1 tsp orange zest
- ¼ cup white sugar
- 1 cup water
- 1 tsp vanilla

LEMON CURD
- 2 eggs
- ½ cup lemon juice
- ¾ cup white sugar
- 3 tablespoons butter

DIRECTIONS

1. **In a saucepan combine all ingredients for cranberry compote**

2. Simmer until mixture thickens
3. For lemon curd add lemon juice, eggs, zest, sugar, water and bring to a boil
4. Remove from heat and fold in butter
5. Layer angel cake with cranberry compote and lemon curd in a parfait glass
6. Garnish with berries
7. When ready remove and serve

RICE BARS

Serves: **12**

Prep Time: **10** Minutes

Cook Time: **60** Minutes

Total Time: **70** Minutes

INGREDIENTS

- 4 cups gluten-free rice cereal
- ¼ cup peanut butter
- 1/3 cup honey
- dash of salt
- 1 tsp vanilla extract
- 2 tablespoons melted chocolate

DIRECTIONS

1. In a bowl combine all ingredients except chocolate
2. Spread the mixture across a prepared pan and press it down into the pan
3. Drizzle melted chocolate over the bars
4. Refrigerate for 50-60 minutes
5. When ready remove and serve

SMOOTHIES

BANANA SMOOTHIE

Serves: **1**

Prep Time: **5** Minutes

Cook Time: **5** Minutes

Total Time: **10** Minutes

INGREDIENTS

- ¼ cup strawberries
- ½ banana
- 1 orange
- 1 cup ice

DIRECTIONS

1. **In a blender place all ingredients and blend until smooth**
2. **Pour smoothie in a glass and serve**

BLUEBERRY DETOX SMOOTHIE

Serves: *1*

Prep Time: *5* Minutes

Cook Time: *5* Minutes

Total Time: *10* Minutes

INGREDIENTS

- 1 banana
- 1 handful of blueberries
- 1 tablespoon coconut oil
- 1 tablespoon hemp seeds
- 1 tablespoon chia seeds
- pinch of cinnamon

DIRECTIONS

1. In a blender place all ingredients and blend until smooth
2. Pour smoothie in a glass and serve

KIDNEY NOURISHING SMOOTHIE

Serves: *1*

Prep Time: *5* Minutes

Cook Time: *5* Minutes

Total Time: *10* Minutes

INGREDIENTS

- ¼ cucumber
- 1 cup blueberries
- 6 oz. coconut water
- 1 tablespoon chia seeds
- 1 tablespoon honey
- ice cubes

DIRECTIONS

1. In a blender place all ingredients and blend until smooth
2. Pour smoothie in a glass and serve

CRANBERRY DETOX SMOOTHIE

Serves: *1*

Prep Time: *5* Minutes

Cook Time: *5* Minutes

Total Time: *10* Minutes

INGREDIENTS

- 1 cup mixed berries
- ½ cup cranberry juice
- ½ avocado
- 1 cup coconut water
- 1 tablespoon chia seeds
- 1 tsp ginger

DIRECTIONS

1. **In a blender place all ingredients and blend until smooth**
2. **Pour smoothie in a glass and serve**

PUMPKIN SMOOTHIE

Serves: **1**

Prep Time: **5** Minutes

Cook Time: **5** Minutes

Total Time: **10** Minutes

INGREDIENTS

- ½ cup pumpkin
- ½ cup coconut milk
- 1 tablespoon chia seeds
- ½ cup coconut water
- 1 tsp honey
- 1 tsp cinnamon
- ¼ tsp nutmeg
- ¼ tsp pumpkin pie spice

DIRECTIONS

1. In a blender place all ingredients and blend until smooth
2. Pour smoothie in a glass and serve

CINNAMON-BLACKBERRY SMOOTHIE

Serves: **1**

Prep Time: **5** Minutes

Cook Time: **5** Minutes

Total Time: **10** Minutes

INGREDIENTS

- 1 cup blackberries
- 1 cup coconut water
- 1 tablespoon chia seeds
- ¼ tsp cinnamon
- 1 handful spinach
- 1 tablespoon honey

DIRECTIONS

1. **In a blender place all ingredients and blend until smooth**
2. **Pour smoothie in a glass and serve**

KALE LIVER DETOX SMOOTHIE

Serves: **1**

Prep Time: **5** Minutes

Cook Time: **5** Minutes

Total Time: **10** Minutes

INGREDIENTS

- 1 cup Kale
- 1 apple
- 1 lemon
- 1-inch ginger
- 1 cup water

DIRECTIONS

1. **In a blender place all ingredients and blend until smooth**
2. **Pour smoothie in a glass and serve**

GREEN DETOX SMOOTHIE

Serves: *1*

Prep Time: *5* Minutes

Cook Time: *5* Minutes

Total Time: *10* Minutes

INGREDIENTS

- 1 cup coconut water
- 1 handful kale
- 1 handful spinach
- 4 stalks celery
- 1 apple
- juice of 1 lemon
- ¼ bunch parsley

DIRECTIONS

1. **In a blender place all ingredients and blend until smooth**
2. **Pour smoothie in a glass and serve**

CLEANSE JUICE

Serves: **1**

Prep Time: **5** Minutes

Cook Time: **5** Minutes

Total Time: **10** Minutes

INGREDIENTS

- 1 beet
- 2 apples
- 2 radishes
- 1 cup kale leaves

DIRECTIONS

1. **In a blender place all ingredients and blend until smooth**
2. **Pour smoothie in a glass and serve**

CARROT AND APPLE MORNING SMOOTHIE

Serves: *1*

Prep Time: *5* Minutes

Cook Time: *5* Minutes

Total Time: *10* Minutes

INGREDIENTS

- 2 apples
- 8 carrots
- ¼ inch ginger
- pinch of cinnamon

DIRECTIONS

1. **In a blender place all ingredients and blend until smooth**
2. **Pour smoothie in a glass and serve**

ENERGY BOOSTING SMOOTHIE

Serves: *1*

Prep Time: *5* Minutes

Cook Time: *5* Minutes

Total Time: *10* Minutes

INGREDIENTS

- 3 stalks celery
- ½ cup parsley
- 1 tsp Spirulina
- juice of ½ lemon

DIRECTIONS

1. **In a blender place all ingredients and blend until smooth**
2. **Pour smoothie in a glass and serve**

PAPAYA SMOOTHIE

Serves: **1**

Prep Time: **5** Minutes

Cook Time: **5** Minutes

Total Time: **10** Minutes

INGREDIENTS

- 2 cups papaya
- 1 tablespoon papaya seeds
- juice of ½ lime
- 1 cup water

DIRECTIONS

1. **In a blender place all ingredients and blend until smooth**
2. **Pour smoothie in a glass and serve**

NO MILK SHAKE

Serves: **1**

Prep Time: **5** Minutes

Cook Time: **5** Minutes

Total Time: **10** Minutes

INGREDIENTS

- ¼ cup pasteurized liquid egg product
- ¼ cup frozen whipped topping
- almond extract
- ¼ cup berries
- ¼ cup apple

DIRECTIONS

1. **In a blender place all ingredients and blend until smooth**
2. **Pour smoothie in a glass and serve**

TURMERIC SMOOTHIE

Serves: *1*

Prep Time: *5* Minutes

Cook Time: *5* Minutes

Total Time: *10* Minutes

INGREDIENTS

- 1 tablespoon turmeric grated
- 1 cup kale
- 1 apple
- 1 cup berries
- 1 cup almond milk

DIRECTIONS

1. **In a blender place all ingredients and blend until smooth**
2. **Pour smoothie in a glass and serve**

BEETROOT DETOX SMOOTHIE

Serves: *1*

Prep Time: *5* Minutes

Cook Time: *5* Minutes

Total Time: *10* Minutes

INGREDIENTS

- 1 cup coconut water
- 1 cup strawberries
- 1 beetroot
- 1 tablespoon chia seeds

DIRECTIONS

1. **In a blender place all ingredients and blend until smooth**
2. **Pour smoothie in a glass and serve**

CARROT & BEETROOT SMOOTHIE

Serves: *1*

Prep Time: *5* Minutes

Cook Time: *5* Minutes

Total Time: *10* Minutes

INGREDIENTS

- 1 beetroot grated
- 1 cup carrot juice
- 1 apple
- 1 tablespoon ginger
- 1/3 cup cilantro
- ¼ cup coconut water

DIRECTIONS

1. In a blender place all ingredients and blend until smooth
2. Pour smoothie in a glass and serve

SPINACH SMOOTHIE

Serves: *1*

Prep Time: *5* Minutes

Cook Time: *5* Minutes

Total Time: *10* Minutes

INGREDIENTS

- 1 cucumber
- 1 cup spinach
- 1 lemon
- 1 cup Swiss chard
- 1 cup water

DIRECTIONS

1. **In a blender place all ingredients and blend until smooth**
2. **Pour smoothie in a glass and serve**

PEACH SMOOTHIE

Serves: **1**

Prep Time: **5** Minutes

Cook Time: **5** Minutes

Total Time: **10** Minutes

INGREDIENTS

- 1 cup ice
- 2 tablespoons powdered egg whites
- ½ cup peaches
- 1 tablespoon sugar

DIRECTIONS

1. **In a blender place all ingredients and blend until smooth**
2. **Pour smoothie in a glass and serve**

GRAPEFRUIT SMOOTHIE

Serves: **1**

Prep Time: **5** Minutes

Cook Time: **5** Minutes

Total Time: **10** Minutes

INGREDIENTS

- 1 grapefruit
- 1 lemon
- 1 cup water
- ½ cucumber
- 1 avocado
- 1 clove garlic
- 1-inch ginger

DIRECTIONS

1. **In a blender place all ingredients and blend until smooth**
2. **Pour smoothie in a glass and serve**

KIWI SMOOTHIE

Serves: **1**

Prep Time: **5** Minutes

Cook Time: **5** Minutes

Total Time: **10** Minutes

INGREDIENTS

- 1 cup almond milk
- 2 kiwi fruits
- 1 banana
- ¼ cup silken tofu
- ¼ cup oats
- ¼ tsp ginger
-

DIRECTIONS

1. In a blender place all ingredients and blend until smooth
2. Pour smoothie in a glass and serve

Made in United States
Troutdale, OR
10/26/2023